YOUR KNOWLEDGE HAS VALUE

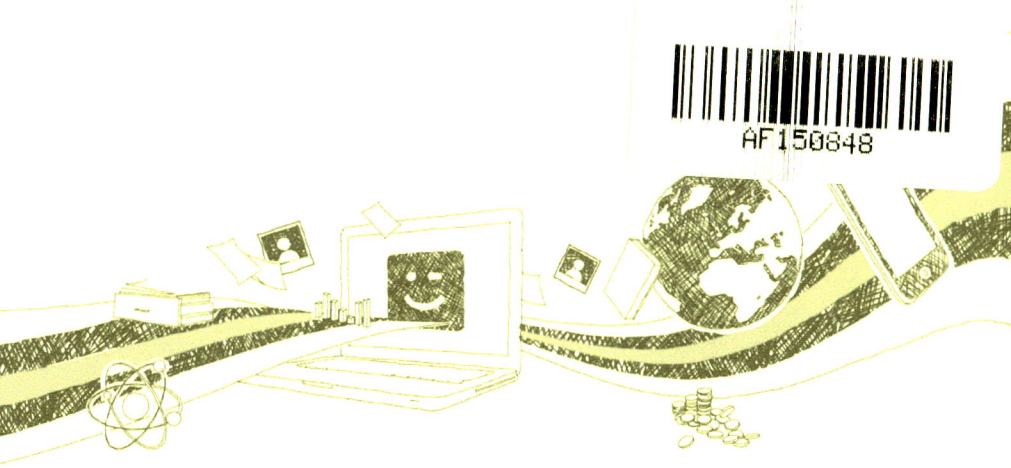

- We will publish your bachelor's and master's thesis, essays and papers

- Your own eBook and book - sold worldwide in all relevant shops

- Earn money with each sale

Upload your text at www.GRIN.com and publish for free

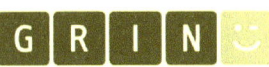

Bibliographic information published by the German National Library:

The German National Library lists this publication in the National Bibliography; detailed bibliographic data are available on the Internet at http://dnb.dnb.de .

Imprint:

Copyright © 2017 GRIN Verlag, Open Publishing GmbH
Print and binding: Books on Demand GmbH, Norderstedt Germany
ISBN: 9783668575493

This book at GRIN:

http://www.grin.com/en/e-book/381246/alternative-methods-of-treating-bipolar-disorder

Patrick Kimuyu

Alternative Methods of treating Bipolar Disorder

GRIN Publishing

GRIN - Your knowledge has value

Since its foundation in 1998, GRIN has specialized in publishing academic texts by students, college teachers and other academics as e-book and printed book. The website www.grin.com is an ideal platform for presenting term papers, final papers, scientific essays, dissertations and specialist books.

Visit us on the internet:

http://www.grin.com/

http://www.facebook.com/grincom

http://www.twitter.com/grin_com

Alternative Methods of Treating Bipolar Disorder

Name: Patrick K. Kimuyu

Table of Content

Alternative Methods of Treating Bipolar Disorder

Introduction

Bipolar disorder has seemingly become one of the most challenging psychiatric illnesses in the U.S and the world at large. Statistics of this disorder were considered relatively insignificant in the past, but recent studies reveal that its prevalence has increased to an alarming level. It is estimated that more than 10 million people in the U.S are suffering from bipolar disorder (Goldberg, 2013[a]). This implies that its burden is relatively high and yet the U.S public healthcare system is facing enormous challenges from non-communicable diseases such as cancer, obesity and its related health conditions. Glick (2004) reports "the socioeconomic and personal burdens of this illness are significant, and the lifetime risk of suicide attempts by patients with bipolar II disorder is high" (p. 27). Therefore, bipolar disorder causes immense personal and socioeconomic burden. World Health Organization ranks bipolar disorder among the top 10 disorders responsible for disability and premature mortality in developing countries. This is probably so because this illness is associated to suicide. Recent studies indicate that 25% to 50% of the population suffering from bipolar disorder has suicide experiences in which women are most affected (Glick, 2004). However, it is worth noting that the prevalence of bipolar disorder is the same among men and women. In addition, it equally in all ethnic groups, socioeconomic classes and races (Goldberg, 2013[a]).

Bipolar disorder is a psychiatric illness in which an individual experiences mania and depression episodes leading to social withdrawal, irritability and extreme sadness. In addition, bipolar mania is characterized with aggressiveness, sexual inappropriateness and exaggerated self-confidence (Goldberg, 2013[a]). As such, its diagnosis and treatment encompasses immense complexity. Glick (2004) states "pharmacotherapeutic management of bipolar disorder is

3

extremely complex, fraught with frequent non-response and resistance to treatment and side effects (p. 31).

However, there are numerous alternatives of treating bipolar disorder, which are more efficient than medication. Therefore, this research paper will discuss alternative methods of dealing with bipolar disorder such as lifestyle changes, nutrition and herbal remedies. It will also provide an overview on medication, and its related side effects to create an understanding of the significance of using alternative treatment approaches.

Common Methods of Dealing with Bipolar Disorder

It is believed that bipolar disorder does not have any cure yet although there are different treatment options. Ordinarily, treatment of bipolar disorder aims at relieving the patient of the signs and symptoms to restore normal mental state. It is believed that maintaining the patients' mental state improves the quality of life. In reality, conventional methods of bipolar disorder treatment are faced with enormous challenges owing to the complexity of the illness. It is reported that mood changes occur even with proper treatment using conventional methods (NIMH, n.d.).

Bipolar disorder is a lifelong illness; thus, it requires long-term continuous treatment for the management of the associated symptoms in which relapse cases are quite common even when medication is successful although this aspect is believed to be enhanced by other mental disorders (NIMH, n.d.). However, alternative remedies have been found to be highly reliable in addressing the challenges caused by medication. Ideally, the most common treatment approaches involve medications with mood stabilizers and antidepressants.

4

Medications and their Effects

From a clinical perspective, medications serve as the only treatment option for managing the symptoms of bipolar disorder. However, misdiagnosis or missed diagnosis renders medication unreliable. In most cases, symptoms of bipolar disorder are overlooked by clinicians leading to immense consequences in bipolar disorder patients. Epidemiological studies indicate that, bipolar disorder is one of the most misdiagnosed depressive disorders with a survey conducted in 2000 showing that 69 percent of bipolar disorder cases were misdiagnosed (Glick, 2004).

Some of the commonly used medications include mood stabilizers, antidepressants and atypical antipsychotics. In practice, mood stabilizers are used as the first choice of treating bipolar disorder, and they are used for a long term to manage mood changes in patients. Historically, mood stabilizers were adopted for clinical use in treating bipolar disorder in 1970 when Lithium was approved by the U.S Food and Drug Agency (FDA). Currently, there is an array of mood stabilizers including Valproic acid, Lamotrigine, Gabapentin and Oxcarbazepine (NIMH, n.d.). However, it is worth noting that, Lithium is used as the most reliable medication for bipolar disorder while the other mood stabilizers including anticonvulsants are used to supplement the latter.

The essence of incorporating alternative treatment options can be explained by the side effects associated with mood stabilizers. For instance, Lithium causes biological changes in the patient's body in which the kidneys and thyroid gland are affected. In most cases, Lithium causes low thyroid function, which is responsible for the rapid cycling observed among people with bipolar disorder, especially women. It is also associated to birth defects; thus, caution is necessary when using Lithium for treating bipolar disorder in pregnant and lactating women

(Goldberg, 2013[b]). In addition, Lithium causes restlessness, acne, muscle pain and unusual discomfort to cold weather. Other side effects include drying of the mouth, indigestion and brittleness of hair or nails (NIMH, n.d.).

Moreover, anticonvulsants are believed to cause unusual mood changes which increase the risk of suicidal behaviors. Therefore, management of bipolar disorder with anticonvulsants requires extensive monitoring of the severity of the principal symptoms to prevent adverse mood changes. As such, treatment of bipolar disorder with anticonvulsants is relatively unreliable because they increase health risks. In general, the most common side effects caused by other mood stabilizers, apart from Lithium, include drowsiness, cold-like symptoms, dizziness, indigestion and headache. These side effects are also experienced by people with bipolar disorder who are under antipsychotic treatment. However, some antipsychotics are associated with blurred vision, skin rashes, sensitivity to sunlight and menstrual problems in women (NIMH, n.d.). On the other hand, antidepressants including Bupropion, Fluoxetine and Sertraline cause nausea, sexual problems and agitation.

Alternative Methods of Treating Bipolar Disorder

It has been found that medications used to treat bipolar disorder causes enormous health consequences in patients. This is so because medication takes a long term leading to residual accumulation of the drug metabolites in the body. These residuals cause biological imbalances in various body organs. For instance, mood stabilizers have been found to cause kidney problems in patients with bipolar disorder. Ordinarily, kidneys serve as sites for excretion of drug metabolites. In the case of Lithium, the functions of kidneys are interrupted by the physiological changes of biological fluids passing through the kidney glomeruli. It is believed that Lithium enhances crystallization of salts in the kidney tubules. As a result, the filtering ability of kidneys

6

is impaired, and this is believed to cause the hardening of the nephrons which are the functional units of the kidneys.

On the other hand, some medications such as anticonvulsants influence an individual's social nature. In most cases, they cause changes in the social behavior which, in turn, triggers suicidal thoughts among people with bipolar disorder. Despite the benefits associated with medications, this treatment approach encompasses fatal consequences. Therefore, it is necessary to adopt other alternatives in treating bipolar disorder. This is seemingly the only way to address the issue of drug toxicity and other psychological consequences caused by medication for bipolar disorder.

Fortunately, there are several remedies for treating the illness which are more efficient than medication although these alternatives have not yet been considered useful by most physicians. It has been found out that lifestyle changes including nutrition, exercise and psychotherapy play a pivotal role in managing the symptoms of bipolar disorder. Social changes such as personal daily routine and social support have also been found to be reliable in dealing with bipolar disorder in most people, even those who are experiencing severe symptoms.

Nutrition

One of the most reliable alternatives of dealing with bipolar disorder is the adoption of a healthy dietary regime. Research studies indicate that diet plays a principal role in determining an individual's health status. In most cases, unhealthy diets such as fad foods are associated with health problems. This is the reason why most non-communicable diseases including obesity and diabetes are believed to be linked to dietary regimes. In the case of bipolar disorder, unhealthy diet leads to the advancement of the symptoms even when proper medication routine is followed.

On the other hand, proper diet has been found to be a reliable remedy for virtually all diseases because a healthy diet supplies the body with all the required nutritional components. It is from the nutritional components that the body forms immune response molecules or fills a deficiency to restore normal biological functioning of the body. Ordinarily, a healthy diet consists of adequate amounts of proteins, carbohydrates, vitamins and minerals. Therefore, people with bipolar disorder are supposed to consume lots of vegetables, whole grains and fruits (Goldberg, 2013[c]). This diet should compose of low amounts of sugar and fats.

Amino Acids for Bipolar Disorder

Despite the fact that there is no specific diet for treating bipolar disorder, some nutritional remedies have been identified which help in reducing the most common symptoms. Currently, there are some nutritional supplements which have been found to be reliable in enhancing brain health and proper functioning of the nervous system. These body components are the most affected by bipolar disorder because its symptoms are related to memory capacity of an individual. Research studies show that nutritional supplements, which contain adequate amounts of amino acids, are useful in treating bipolar disorder in people. Some of the most significant amino acids include lecithin, choline, taurine, inositol, phenylalanine and gaba-amino butyric acid (GABA). Moreover, tyrosine, S-adenosyl-methionine (SAME) and methionine have been found to relieve people with bipolar disorder of the associated symptoms (Haggerty, 2008[a]).

In practice, methionine and its metabolites including S-adenosyl-methionine have been used for the treatment of depression. Methionine is an antioxidant amino acid, which exerts energizing effects in depressed individuals. Its metabolite has also been used in the treatment of depression and arthritis in Europe, and its use has now become popular in the United States after its introduction in 1999. On the other hand, tyrosine and phenylalanine boost the production of neurotransmitters, primarily dopamine and norepinephrine which are responsible for the maintenance of stable mood and mental activity. In addition, these two amino acids have been found to promote optimal functioning of the thyroid gland among people with bipolar disorder (Haggerty, 2008[a]). As such, they counter the side effects of mood stabilizers, primarily Lithium which has been found to cause low functioning of the thyroid gland.

Gaba-amino butyric acid acts as a neurotransmitter, and it can be used to treat nervous tension, anxiety and the racing thoughts associated with insomnia. As such, it acts more or less the same way as most anticonvulsants such as Depakote and Gabapentin. However, it is worth noting that, GABA does not cause adverse health consequences observed with the use of mood stabilizers. On the other hand, choline and lecithin are reliable in stabilizing mood because they enhance mental alertness and other brain processes such as learning and memory. Recent studies indicate that lecithin is useful in treating bipolar mania because it depresses mood. It has also been found out that choline enhances regulatory functions in the brain and boost emotional control (Haggerty, 2008[a]).

Other amino acids, which are reliable in treating bipolar disorder, are taurine and inositol. Taurine is believed to enhance efficient electrical activity of the brain; thus, it prevents the occurrence of mood swings in people with bipolar disorder. It has also been found to be useful for patients with rapid cycler episodes because it has anti-seizure capabilities. However, it is worth noting that, this amino acid records appreciable results when administered in a daily range of 500 to 1000 mg per day. Studies indicate that people with bipolar disorder that use doses exceeding 1000 mg per day experiences unusual EEG activity (Haggerty, 2008[a]). On the other hand, inositol helps in preventing nerve damage and boosts the production of serotonin which is responsible for the maintenance of stable mood and sleep. Therefore, it can be used to treat depression in people with bipolar disorder.

Minerals for Bipolar Disorder

A healthy diet should contain adequate amounts of minerals. Ordinarily, minerals are required in the body in small quantities; therefore, people with bipolar disorder should ensure that their food sources are rich in minerals. For instance, vegetables, fruits and whole grains contain considerable amounts of essential mineral elements. However, the quantity of these minerals depends on the source of food. In most cases, food crops growing in mineral deficient soils contain inadequate quantities of minerals. As a result, supplementation with the required quantities is necessary. However, it is worth noting that, not all minerals are useful in treating bipolar symptoms. Instead, only some few mineral elements have been found to alleviate bipolar symptoms. Some of the most reliable minerals include manganese, calcium, zinc and magnesium.

Calcium serves as one of the most essential minerals in the body because it is involved in an array of biological functions. Apart from its function in bone formation, calcium helps in the production of neurotransmitters such as calmodulin which enhance the functioning of the nervous system. On the other hand, magnesium works almost the same way as calcium in regulating the functioning of the nervous system through promoting the transmission of impulses. As such, it can be used to treat anxiety and insomnia. In most cases, deficiency of magnesium lowers seizure threshold, especially under stressful and hot weather conditions (Haggerty, 2008[b]). Therefore, supplementation alleviates insomnia in people with bipolar disorder.

Manganese and zinc are required in the body in trace amounts, which can be obtained from mineral rich diet. However, some diets do not contain the required daily requirements leading to deficiencies related to these minerals. In practice, deficiency of manganese causes memory problems, fatigue and irritability even in people who are not suffering from bipolar disorder. Therefore, its deficiency in bipolar patients worsens the disorder symptoms, and these symptoms can be alleviated through supplementation with the required daily mineral requirements. On the other hand, zinc deficiency causes mental disturbances, and this complicates bipolar symptoms (Haggerty, 2008[b]). Therefore, people with bipolar disorder require adequate quantities of zinc, either from the diet or supplementation to prevent its deficiency symptoms.

Chromium picolinate has also been found to be reliable in treating bipolar symptoms. It controls carbohydrate and sugar craving which is common among bipolar patients (Haggerty, 2008[b]). Therefore, it can be used to replace mood stabilizer such Depakote because this drug bears adverse side effects compared to chromium picolinate.

Vitamins for Bipolar Disorder

Treatment of bipolar symptoms involves the utilization of different vitamins. Studies indicate that people with bipolar disorder exhibit differences from healthy people in the way vitamins metabolism occur in the body. Ordinarily, vitamins deficiency lowers immune capabilities of an individual's body; thus, making it unable to fight pathogens. However, it is worth noting that different vitamins serve different functions in the body. For instance, vitamin B complexes and folic acid play a significant role in alleviating anxiety, depression and fatigue, and these are the most common bipolar symptoms. Therefore, dietary sources for bipolar people

11

should contain adequate quantities of folic acid and vitamin B complexes which include thiamin (vitamin B-1), cobalamin (vitamin B-12), vitamin E and pyridoxine (B-6).

Thiamin has been found to be useful in alleviating irritability and anxiety in people with bipolar disorder. In addition, it prevents tingling of the extremities and blood circulatory problems which are experienced by bipolar patients. Vitamin B-6 plays the same role in treating bipolar symptoms, but it also deals with motion sickness and other symptoms, especially those related to premenstrual conditions among women. On the other hand, vitamin B-12 enhances food metabolism in the body; thus, preventing fatigue. This vitamin is commonly found in adequate quantities in animal products. Therefore, bipolar vegetarians are likely to experience vitamin B-12 deficiency unless supplementation is provided. Moreover, vitamin E helps in reducing the frequency of seizures in bipolar patients more or less the same as it is the case in epilepsy. However, it is worth noting that, anticonvulsants, which are used as medication for bipolar disorder depletes vitamin E in the body, and this is probably the reason as to why seizures are quite persistent in bipolar patients who are under anticonvulsant treatment. On the other hand, folic acid has been found to be reliable in counteracting the side effects of anticonvulsants (Haggerty, 2008ᶜ).

Moreover, Omega-3 fatty acids are reliable in dealing with bipolar symptoms. From a biological approach, omega-3 fatty acids form essential components of brain cells. As such, they enhance brain functioning through facilitating efficient impulse transmission in the brain. They have also been found to boost memory. Therefore, bipolar patients should ensure there are adequate quantities in their diet for their brain health. Some of the richest sources of omega-3 fatty acids include fish oil, especially salmon fish, avocado and almond oil. Currently, omega-3 fatty acids supplements are available in the market, so bipolar patients can get adequate supplies of these oils through supplementation in case they do not consume omega-3 rich diets.

Alcohol and Caffeine

Despite the enormous benefits provided by diet, some dietary components cause adverse health consequences to bipolar patients. For instance, alcohol consumption and caffeine have been found to enhance the advancement of bipolar symptoms.

Caffeine has been found to cause disruption of sleep cycles in people with bipolar disorder. Ordinarily, impairment of sleep cycles leads to hypomania and mania attacks; thus, caffeinated substances such as coffee are not suitable for bipolar patients. Caffeine has also been found to cause anxiety and panicking in bipolar patients, and this causes insomnia. Moreover, research studies indicate that caffeine increases the risk of suicide. Margolis (2010) reports "a 2009 study uncovered an alarming finding by showing that, drinking coffee appears to increase suicide attempts among bipolar patients" (par. 1).

Effects of drug Abuse and Bipolar Disorder

It is advisable for people with bipolar disorder to avoid alcohol consumption and other drug abuse. In practice, alcohol consumption and drug abuse worsen bipolar symptoms, especially in bipolar patients with alcoholism predisposing genes (McManamy, 2012). In most cases, substance abuse causes dual diagnosis, which is relatively difficult to treat. It is believed that the co-occurring disorders interact synergistically to produce the overall effect observed in co-morbidity patients. In some cases, the presence of untreated mental health issue enhances the severity of the substance abuse problem. However, the advancement of the substance abuse problems causes an increase in the impact of the mental health disorder; thus, causing unprecedented complication. For instance, drug or alcohol abuse has been found to increase mental health disorders, especially with regard to depression.

However, it is worth to understand the basis of the co-occurring disorders and their relationship among individuals. As such, a nurse has to understand which of the co-occurring disorders appears first or which of the two problems influence the onset of the other. Clinical research indicates that, most people with mental health problems tend to be addicted to drugs. However, it is worth noting that, neither substance abuse nor depression or anxiety influence the cause of each other, even though, these two problems are linked. In most cases, symptoms of depression are often self-medicated using drugs or alcohol because they seem to relieve individuals of depression. However, the mental health problem may become worse, owing to the side effects of substance abuse. In such circumstances, the mental health disorder can be viewed to as the cause of substance abuse (Saisan, Segal & Smith, 2013).

On the other hand, the risk of mental health disorders has been found to be increased by substance abuse. Ordinarily, interplay of different factors such as genetic, social and environmental factors is believed to be the cause of mental health disorders, but substance abuse enhances the strength of the underlying risk factors to establish the mental health disorder. In such a case, substance abuse can be viewed to as the cause of the mental health problem because the other underlying risk factors are not manifested during the onset of the mental health problem.

Moreover, the symptoms of most mental health problems, including depression are believed to be worsened by substance abuse. For instance, alcohol or drug abuse among individuals with mental health problems triggers new symptoms or increase the severity of the existing bipolar symptoms. In regard to medication, alcohol or drug abuse influences the impact of medication with anti-depressants, mood stabilizers and anti-anxiety pills. In general, substance abuse reduces the efficacy of medication administered to address mental health disorders such as depression (Saisan, Segal & Smith, 2013). In general, substance abuse interferes with the management of mental health problems, leading to unprecedented complications among the affected individuals. This is so because; bipolar disorder promotes the development of alcohol abuse tendencies (Goldberg, 2013[b]).

Exercise and Bipolar Disorder

Exercise has also been found to be helpful in dealing with bipolar symptoms. Ordinarily, physical exercise enhances mental functioning and relieves tension. Goldberg (2013[c]) reports that regular exercise plays a fundamental role in improving mood and sleep. It also promotes blood flow in the brain and other body organs leading to the efficient supply of nutrients to the body tissues. However, it is worth noting that, physical exercise does not mean someone must engage in strenuous exercise to achieve its health benefits. In fact, taking a walk along paths in the neighborhood for about 15 minutes is adequate, but cycling is more beneficial than walking. It is also reported that, aerobic exercise helps in treating depression in bipolar patients because it reduces bipolar episodes. Therefore, it is advisable for bipolar patients to maintain a daily routine that allows them to engage in exercise for at least five times a week (Smith, 2013).

Yoga for Bipolar Disorder

Yoga is also useful in treating bipolar symptoms because it involves physical exercise emotional elements and meditation. Ideally, yoga in bipolar patients helps to alleviate anxiety and stress because it enhances the relaxation of the body. It also promotes physical fitness owing to its ability to boost flexibility and balance. Watt (2012) states "Exercise, along with adequate sleep and a nutritious diet, forms the basis of general good health, which can only help someone dealing with a chronic illness like bipolar disorder" (par. 3).

Sleep and Bipolar Disorder

Alternative treatment of bipolar disorder can also involve a strict sleep schedule to prevent insomnia episodes. Ordinarily, sleep patterns of an individual serve as significant determinants of serotonin levels in the body. In bipolar patients, sleep plays a significant role in preventing mania. Ideally, patients should maintain a normal sleep schedule that allows them to have adequate sleep because little sleep has been found to trigger mania. In contrast, prolonged sleep influences mood swings, which are one of the most disturbing conditions of bipolar disorder. Therefore, bipolar patients can prevent the occurrence of mania and mood swing through sleeping and waking up at the same time on a daily basis without changing the sleep schedule (Smith, 2013).

In general, sleep disturbances causes several consequences. For instance, it impairs the quality of life by causing negative psychosocial, economic, health and occupational impacts. It also contributes to cases of relapse in bipolar disorder. In most cases, prodromes of episodes are observed in bipolar patients who experience sleep disturbances, and this increases their chances of experiencing mania or depression. Moreover, sleep disturbances impair the regulation of the neural system (Gershon, Talbot & Harvey, 2009). Therefore, bipolar patients can address all the problems associated with sleep disturbances through observing strict sleep schedule.

Cognitive-Behavioral Therapy

Cognitive-behavioral therapy has also been found to be a reliable alternative in treating bipolar symptoms. In CBT, patients with depression and anxiety are guided to change their negative thoughts. It also helps patients to recognize bipolar symptoms and initiate appropriate

16

behavioral changes before they advance to adverse situations. Ideally, CBT enables bipolar patients to cope with depression through offsetting negative mood (Simon, 2013).

Conclusion

In a brief conclusion, bipolar disorder has been found to be causing an enormous burden to the global healthcare systems. In the U.S, bipolar disorder is quite prevalence with an estimation of 10 million people suffering from the disorder. This is probably the reason as to why the prevalence of mental health illnesses is high, although substance abuse accounts for the highest percentage.

Over the years, medication has always been considered as the only reliable approach of dealing with the disorder. Some of the medications used for the treatment of bipolar disorder include mood stabilizers, anticonvulsants and atypical antipsychotics. However, this illness encompasses complexity which makes difficult to treat. Therefore, proper treatment involves a combination of different drugs, usually over a long-term. As a result, medication causes adverse side effects even when proper treatment is followed; thus, reducing health outcomes.

Surprisingly, all the challenges encountered in treating bipolar symptoms with medications can be solved with the use of alternative remedies, primarily lifestyle changes. Some of the most reliable alternatives of treating bipolar disorder include a healthy diet, exercise and personal daily routine. It has been found out that lifestyle changes combined with Cognitive-Behavioral Therapy enables bipolar patients to enjoy quality life without medications. Therefore, alternative treatments should be considered relevant in dealing with bipolar symptoms because they are more reliable than medical treatment approaches.

References

Gershon, A., Talbot, L. & Harvey, A. G. (2009). Sleep Disturbance in Bipolar Disorder. *Clin Psychol (New York),* 16(2): 256–277. Retrieved from National Health Insitute: http://www.ncbi.nlm.nih.gov/pmc/articles/PMC3321357/

Glick, I. D. (2004). *Undiagnosed Bipolar Disorder: New Syndromes and New Treatments.* Retrieved from National Health Institute: http://www.ncbi.nlm.nih.gov/pmc/articles/PMC427610/#__ffn_sectitle

Goldberg, J. (2013[a]). *Bipolar Disorder, Who's At Risk?* Retrieved from WebMD: http://www.webmd.com/bipolar-disorder/guide/bipolar-disorder-whos-at-risk

Goldberg, J. (2013[b]). *Lithium for Bipolar Disorder.* Retrieved from WebMD: http://www.webmd.com/bipolar-disorder/bipolar-disorder-lithium?page=2

Goldberg, J. (2013[c]). *Living Healthy with Bipolar.* Retrieved from WebMD: http://www.webmd.com/bipolar-disorder/guide/living-healthy-life-with-bipolar

Goldberg, J. (2013[d]). *Bipolar Disorder and Foods To Avoid.* Retrieved from WebMD: http://www.webmd.com/bipolar-disorder/guide/bipolar-diet-foods-to-avoid?page=3

Haggerty, J. (2008[a]). *Nutritional Supplements for Bipolar Disorder.* Retrieved from Everydayhealth: http://www.everydayhealth.com/bipolar-disorder/bipolar-treatments/supplements.aspx

Haggerty, J. (2008[b]) *Minerals for Bipolar Disorder.* Retrieved from Everyday health: http://www.everydayhealth.com/bipolar-disorder/bipolar-treatments/minerals.aspx

Haggerty, J. (2008[c]) *Vitamins for Bipolar Disorder.* Retrieved from Everyday health: http://www.everydayhealth.com/bipolar-disorder/bipolar-treatments/vitamins.aspx

Margolis, R. E. (2013). *Caffeine and Bipolar Disorder.* Retrieved from Livestrong:

http://www.livestrong.com/article/90028-caffeine-bipolar-disorder/

McManamy, J. (2012). *The Cruel Double Whammy: Bipolar and Alcohol or Drug Abuse.*

Retrieved from Health Central:

http://www.healthcentral.com/bipolar/c/15/150631/bipolar-alcohol-drug/2

NIMH. (n.d.). *Bipolar Disorder?* Retrieved from National Institute of Mental Health:

http://www.nimh.nih.gov/health/topics/bipolar-disorder/index.shtml

Saisan, J., Segal, J. & Smith, M. (2013). *Substance Abuse & Mental Health.* Retrieved from

Helpguide.org: http://www.helpguide.org/mental/dual_diagnosis.htm

Simon, H. (2013, November 28). *Psychotherapy and Lifestyle Changes.* Retrieved from New

York Times: http://www.nytimes.com/health/guides/disease/bipolar-

disorder/psychotherapy-and-lifestyle-changes.html

Smith, M. (2013). *Bipolar Support and Self-Help.* Retrieved from Helpguide.org:

http://www.helpguide.org/mental/bipolar_disorder_self_help.htm

Watt, A. (2012). *Yoga for Bipolar Disorder.* Retrieved from Healthline:

http://www.healthline.com/health/bipolar-disorder/yoga

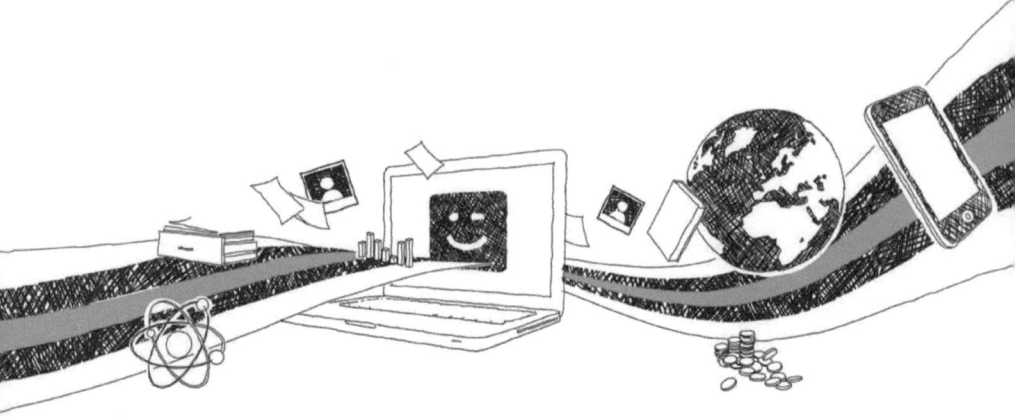
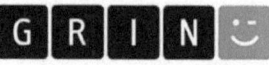